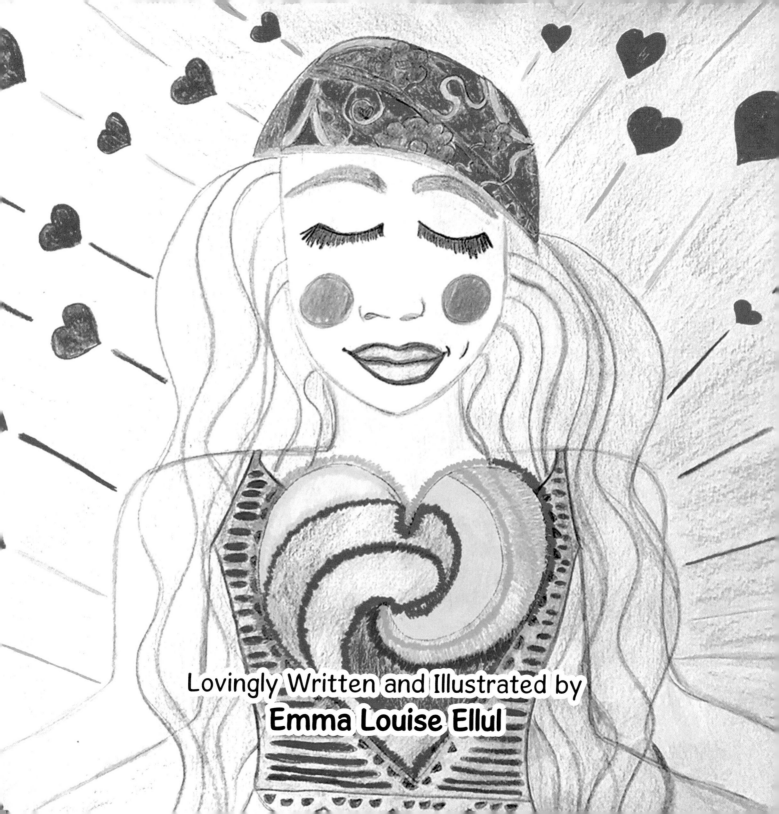

Lovingly Written and Illustrated by
Emma Louise Ellul

Balboa Press books may be ordered through booksellers or by contacting:

Balboa Press
A Division of Hay House
1663 Liberty Drive
Bloomington, IN 47403
www.balboapress.com.au
1 (877) 407-4847

Because of the dynamic nature of the Internet, any web addresses or links contained in this book may have changed since publication and may no longer be valid. The views expressed in this work are solely those of the author and do not necessarily reflect the views of the publisher, and the publisher hereby disclaims any responsibility for them.

Any people depicted in stock imagery provided by Getty Images are models, and such images are being used for illustrative purposes only.
Certain stock imagery © Getty Images.

ISBN: 978-1-5043-1999-7 (sc)
978-1-5043-2000-9 (e)

Print information available on the last page.

Balboa Press rev. date: 05/16/2022

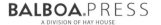

Feel the Love

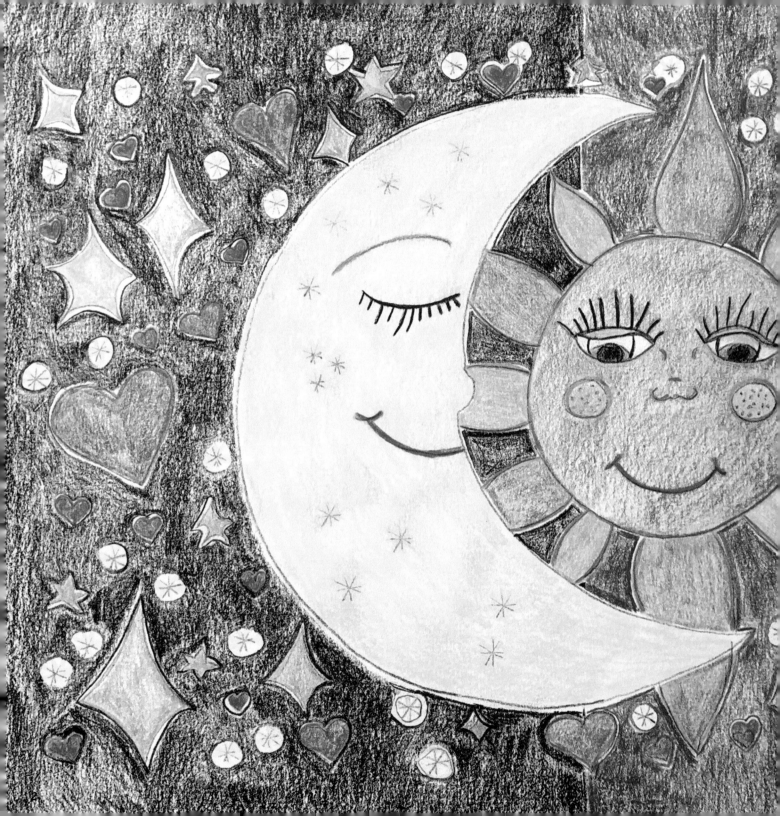

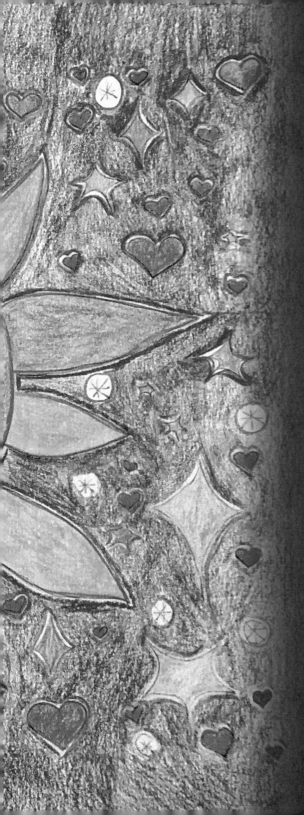

I AM SAFE.

It's time to dream my
precious one....

Today has been and
tomorrow will come.

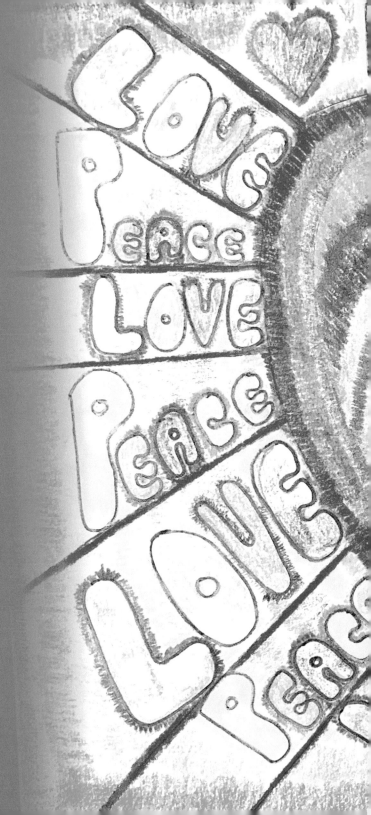

I RELAX AND LET GO.

What kind of a day
have you had today?

Well however it was....
with peace and love
send it on it's way...

4

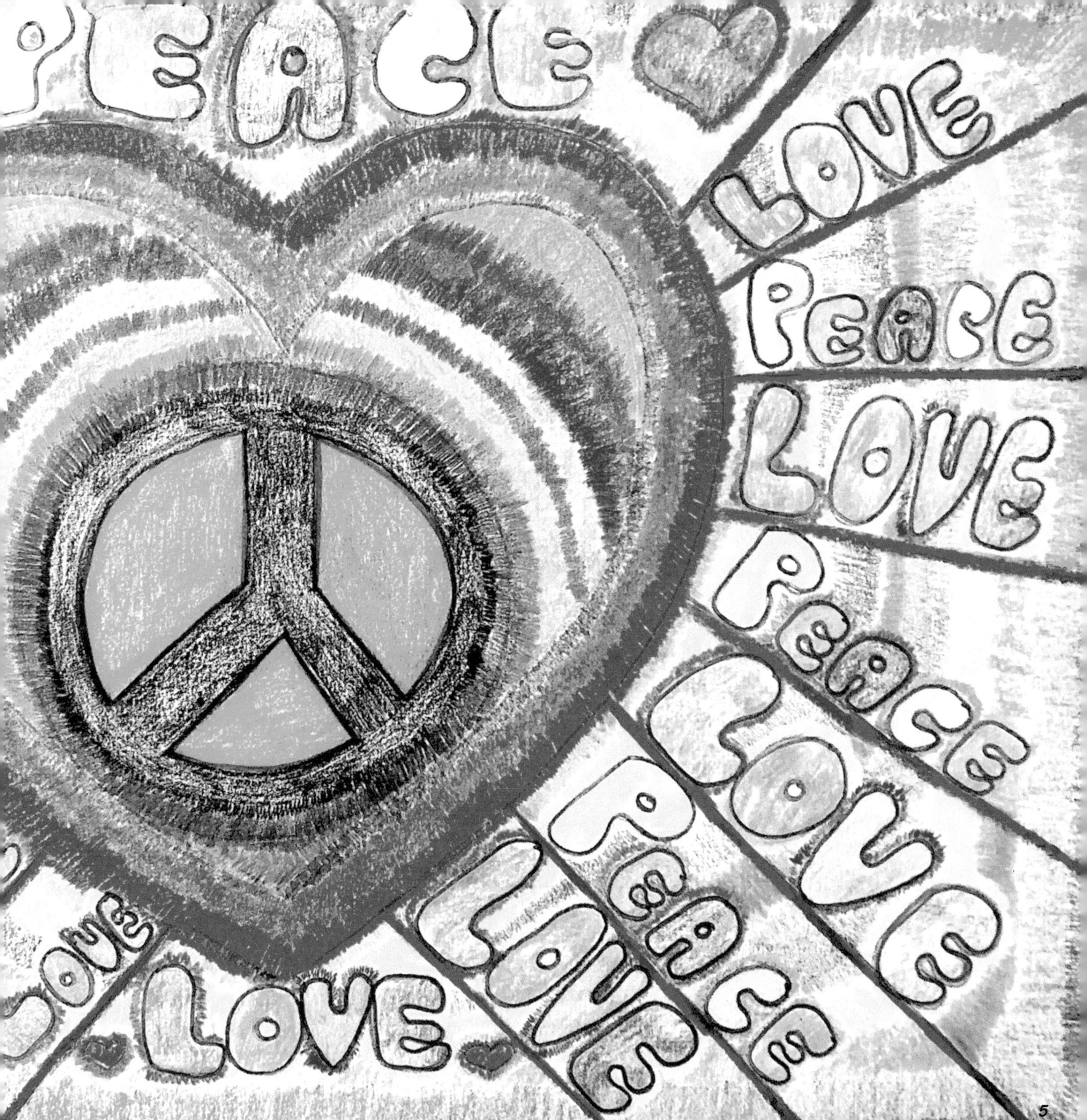
PEACE
LOVE
PEACE
LOVE
PEACE
LOVE
PEACE
LOVE
LOVE
LOVE

I AM CALM AND RELAXED.

Whatever has been just let it go....

Breathe in through your nose......

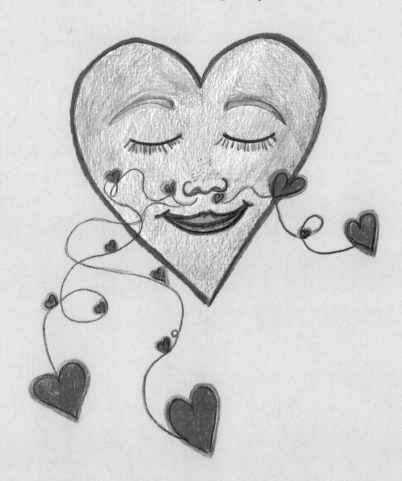

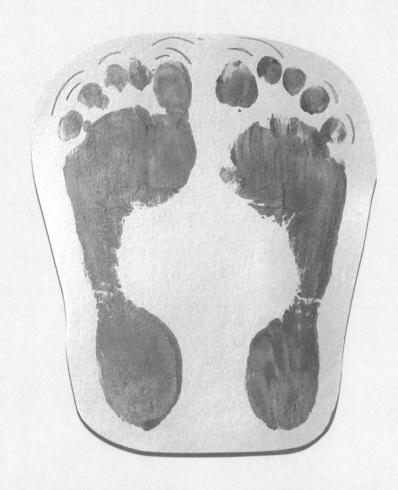

and wiggle your toes.......
(wiggle wiggle wiggle)

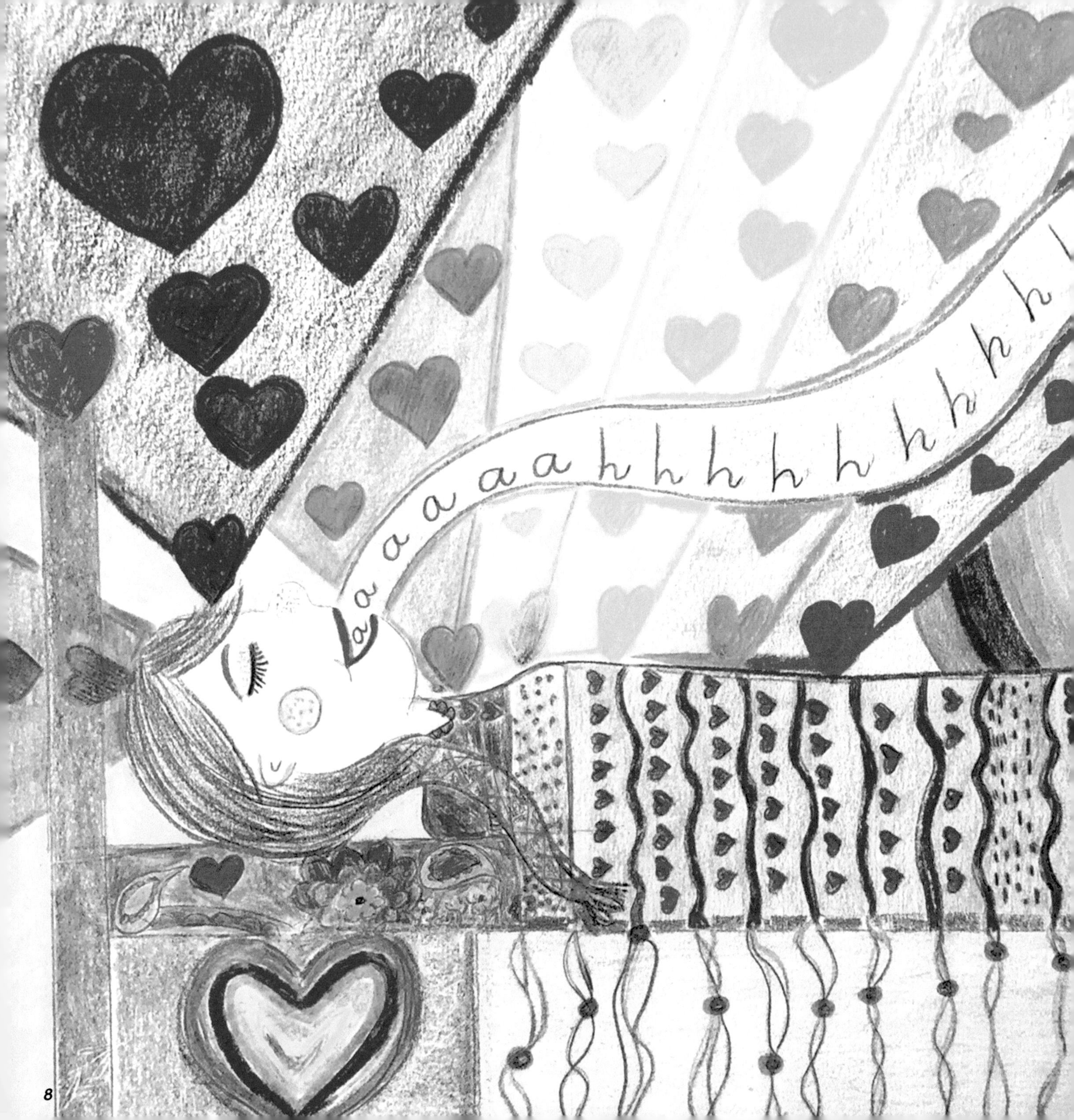
Laaaaaahhhhhhhhhhh

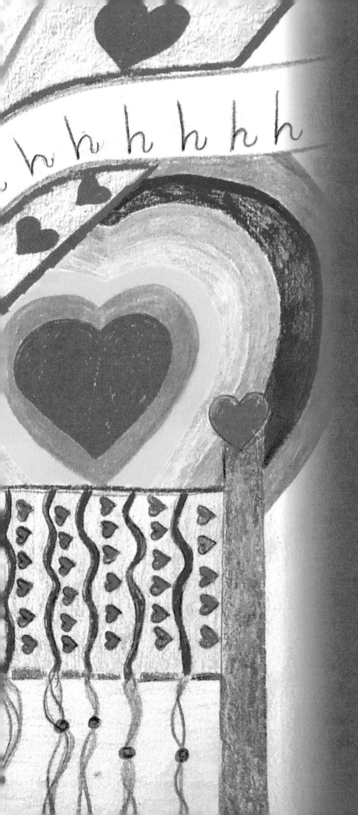

IT FEELS GOOD TO RELAX MY BODY.

Now roll your head
from side to side,

Shrug your shoulders
and let out a sigh,
aaaahhhhhhhh.

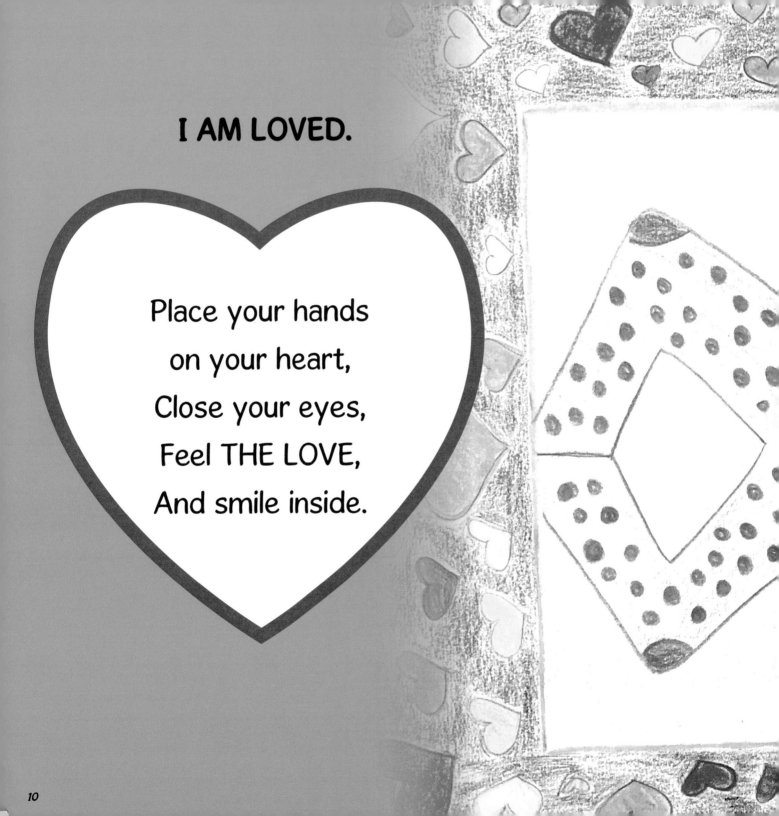

I AM LOVED.

Place your hands
on your heart,
Close your eyes,
Feel THE LOVE,
And smile inside.

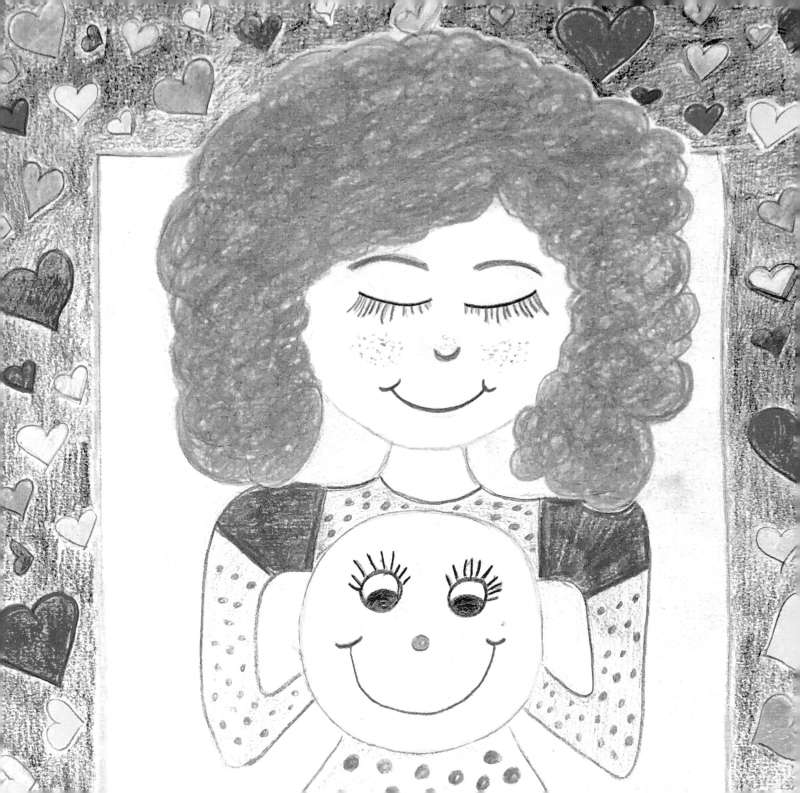

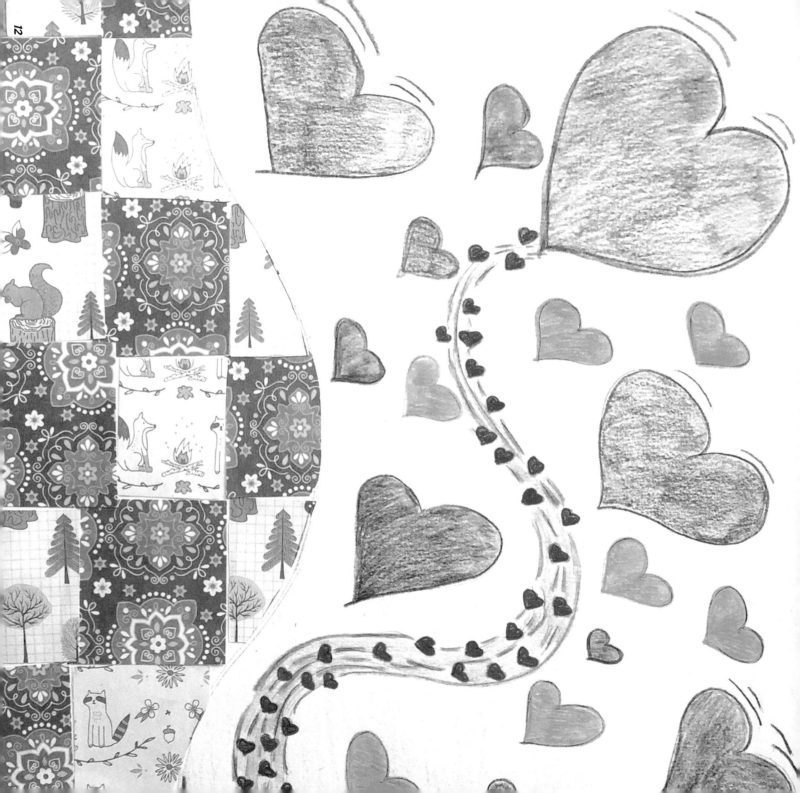

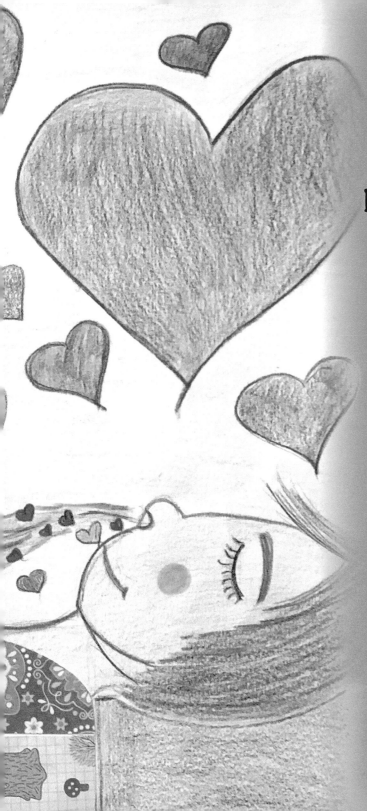

I SLEEP DEEPLY TONIGHT.

Breathe into your belly,

Nice and deep (breathe in
now through your nose),

Now breathe it out,
(through your mouth),

It's nearly your time to
sleep.......... AAaaahhhhh

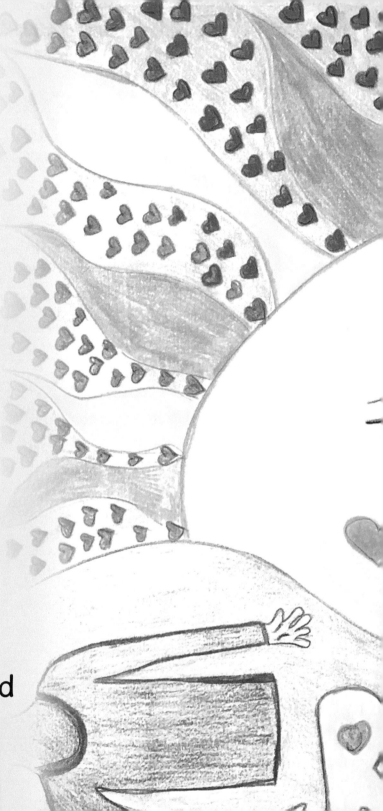

MY BODY IS SO RELAXED NOW.

Rest your arms
my dear child,

Feel them loose and
limp and tired.

Relax your legs,

Your knees

And feet.

You've done your best and
this day is complete.

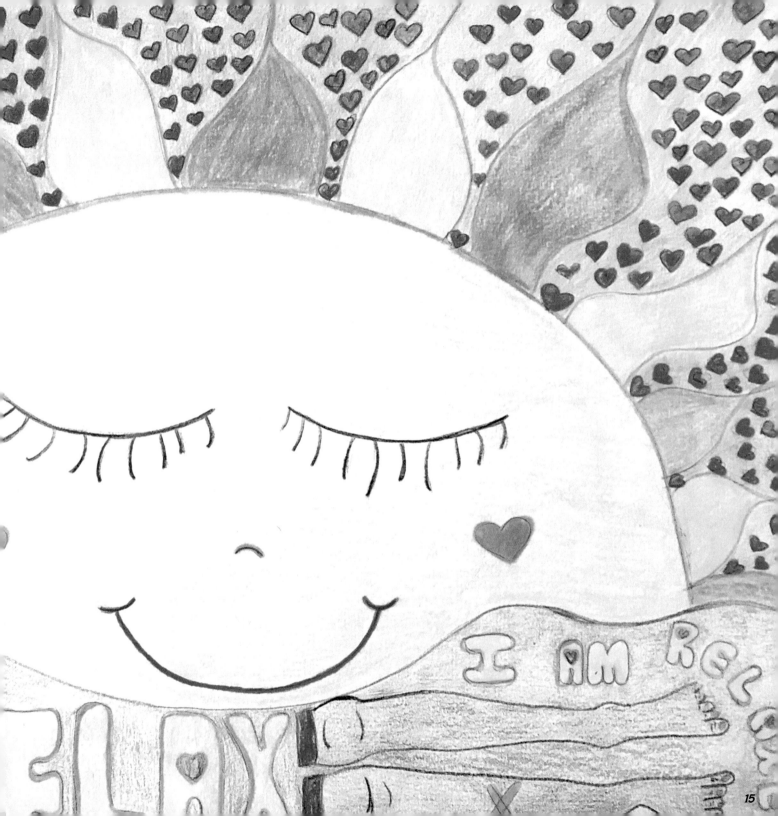

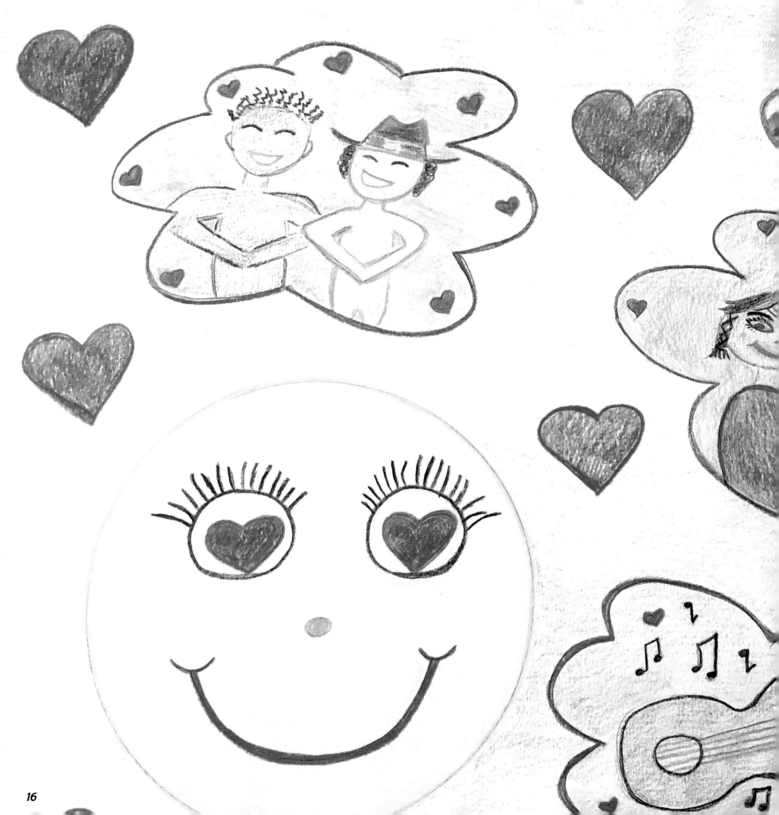

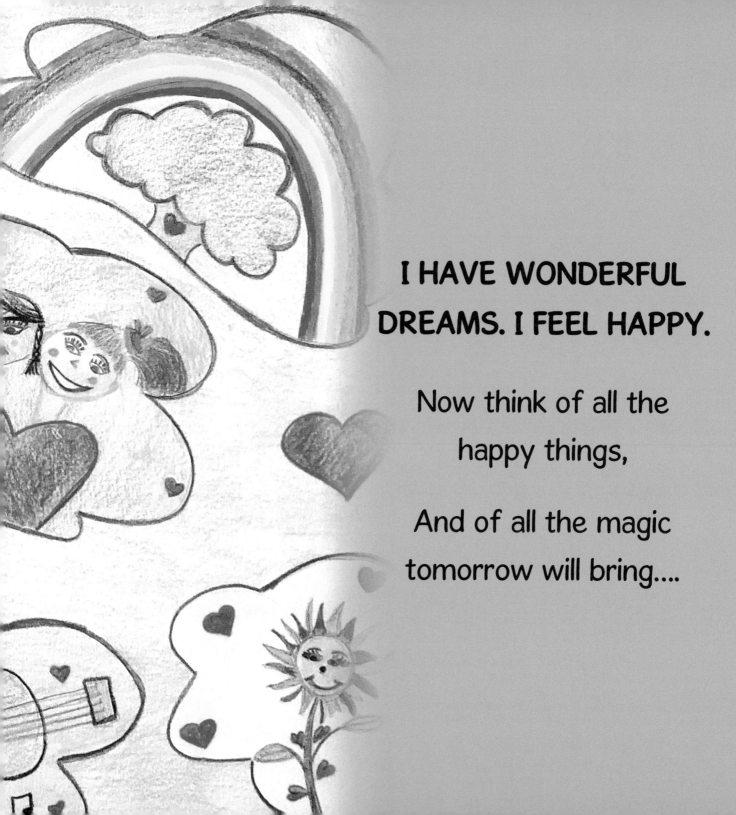

I HAVE WONDERFUL DREAMS. I FEEL HAPPY.

Now think of all the happy things,

And of all the magic tomorrow will bring....

I AM AMAZING.

Now drift, and rest, and sleep, and dream....

Of all the amazing things that you can be.

Be Kind, Be Brave, Be Strong, Be wise...

And life will surely be full of wonder and surprise.

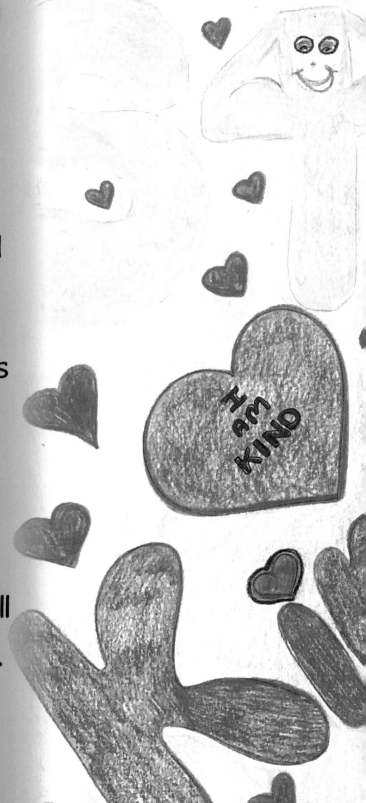

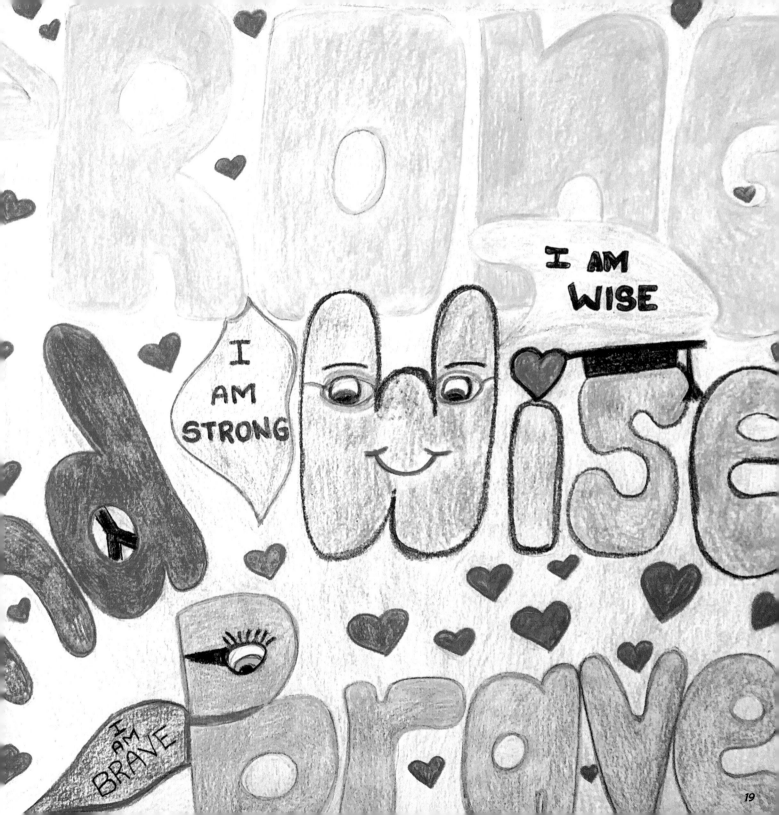

19

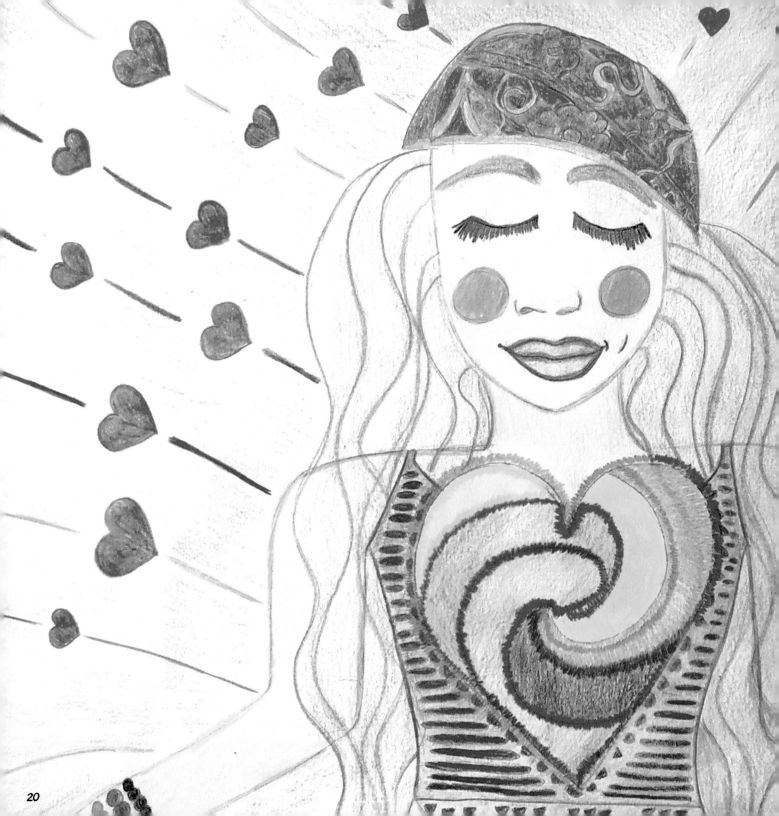

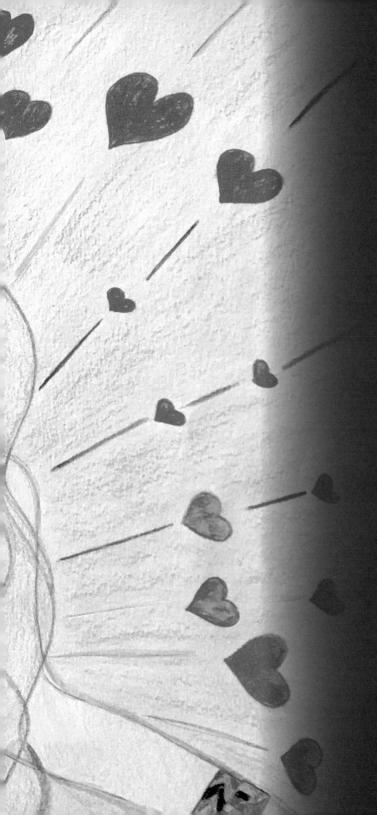

I AM BLESSED.

You are Special, Sacred,
a one of a kind.

And inside of YOU, all you
need, you will find.......

I FEEL PEACEFUL.

Just relax and let
yourself go,

And as you sleep your
soul will grow,

And when you wake,
you will know,

All there is you
need to know.

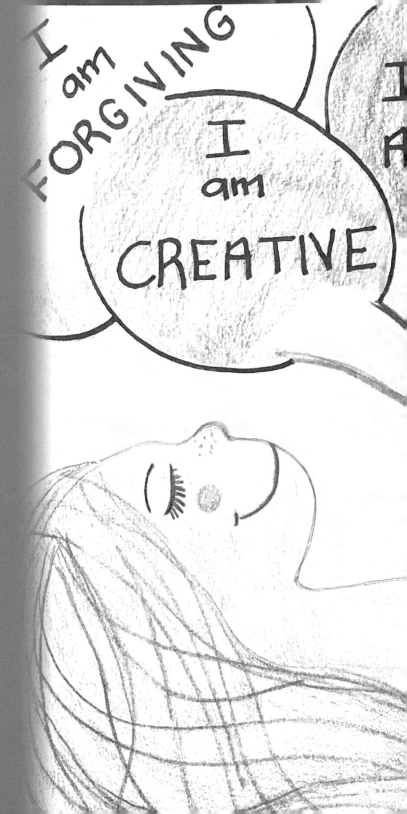

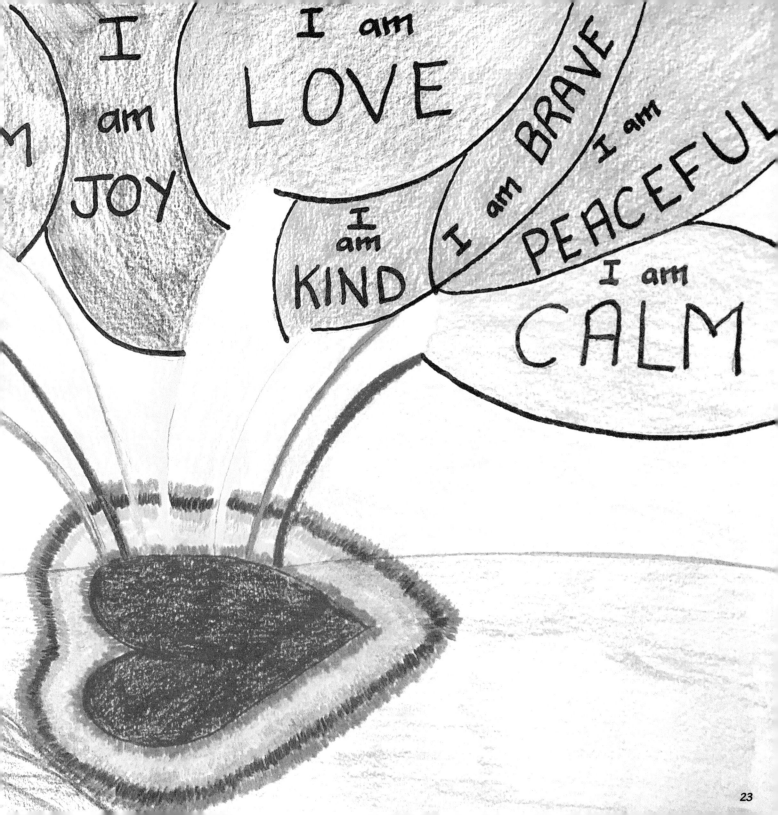

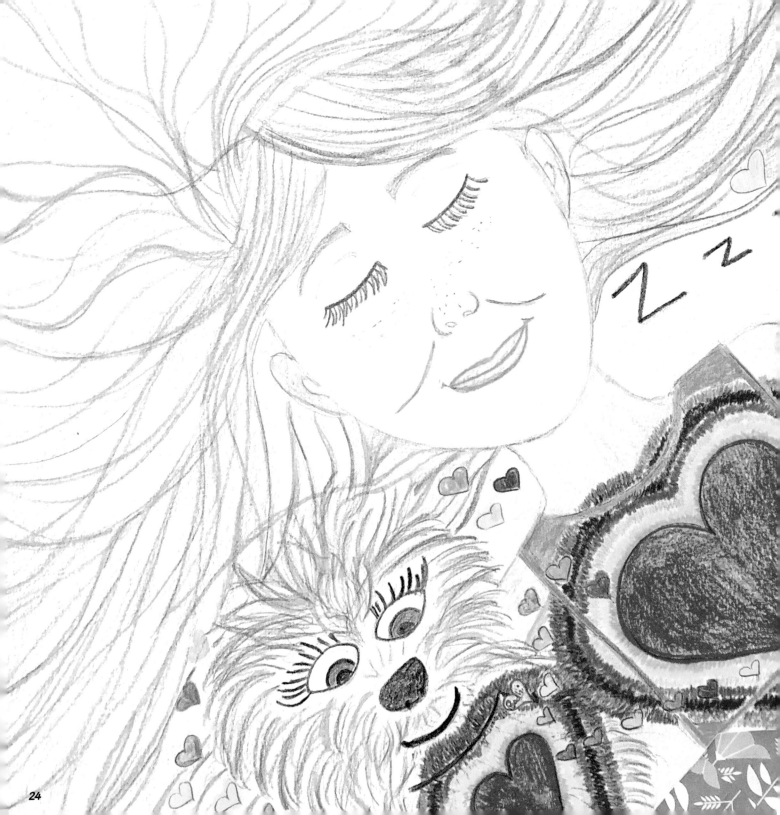

I AM LOVED.

Breathe into your belly,

Nice and deep (breathe in
now through your nose),

Now breathe it out,
(through your mouth),

Goodnight my love,
It's time to sleep.

AFFIRMATIONS

(read gently in a soft, peaceful voice as
your child is drifting off to sleep)

You are going to have the most beautiful sleep tonight.
You will dream of wonderful things. You are always
safe and protected. You are so loved. I love you. You
are perfect exactly as you are. People love being
around you. You are full of joy. I love everything about
you. The world is a better place because you are in
it. You are understanding and kind. You are helpful
and loving. You are forgiving. You are beautiful inside
and out. You are confident and creative. You deserve

all things good in your life. You deserve to be happy and loved. Every day in every way you are getting better and better. You are healthy and happy. You are valued and appreciated. You make wise choices. You are a good learner, and you remember things easily. You are kind and caring. You easily stand up for yourself and others. You are brave, and calmly face new experiences. You are loved and supported in all ways. You are a blessing. You are calm and peaceful. You are loved.

MY FAVOURITE FEEL GOOD WORDS
(write them here, these next few
pages are just for YOU)

THINGS THAT I AM GREATFUL FOR

THINGS THAT I LOVE ABOUT ME!

A HAPPY PICTURE

Dear Parents and Care Givers, THis LOVING Bedtime book teaches our children the power of the breath, how to relax their bodies, and introduces the Power of Affirmations.

It helps them learn how to breathe consciously. Be present. And to focus their attention on different areas of their bodies to relax.

Not just at bedtime, but anytime!

THey learn to let go of 'this day', and know they get a brand new day tomorrow to do things differently.

The Affirmations throughout this book will begin them on their journey of ' the power of their thoughts and words.'

They will begin to release worries, fears, and anxieties, as these feelings/emotions switch to feelings of love, security, safety, feeling valued, hopeful , empowered, and looking forward to their tomorrow.

The Affirmations will soak into their subconscious overnight, and you will very quickly notice your child move into more moments of love, joy, hope and excitement.

I truly hope this book brings you some support, and positivity on this neverending parenting journey.

Love Em x

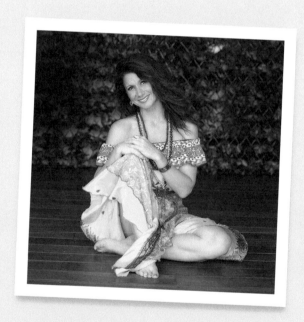

Printed in the United States
by Baker & Taylor Publisher Services